Shift
The Business
Side of Massage

Kamillya Hunter

Shift: The Business Side Of Massage

Copyright © 2018 Kamillya Hunter

Cover designed by: www.herbookbar.com

Image by: Elka Photography

ISBN: 9781723839160

CONTENTS

INTRODUCTION

Creating a practice that can function and thrive independent of you is a concept many solo massage therapists struggle with. Although the struggle is not unique to massage therapists, this type of service is extremely personal. Because of that, many therapists believe that in order to maintain consistent high level standards and offer the best care, they must be the ones to deliver each service. That belief is one of the driving forces behind the reason many massage therapists start their own business. As owner, you are able to control the entire client's experience.

When I polled a closed Facebook group. Massage and Spa Business Details That Matter, the most common reasons therapists started their own practice were: control, more money, flexible schedule, better working conditions, and distance from a bad employer. The responses were not surprising. Though the sample size was relatively small, I would argue these reasons rank pretty high for why anyone chooses to start a business. Regardless of why, an overwhelming amount of them admit they are not sure how to build and manage a business.

As entrepreneurs, we have a tendency to focus on exciting details of starting and growing a business. Those details tend to include marketing collateral (business cards, logos, websites, etc.). Massage entrepreneurs stretch that focus to treatment room décor, adding advanced modalities to their arsenal of skills, and fancy tools that only other massage therapists would recognize.

No one will disagree that those are important components of a massage practice. You may know how to provide an amazing service and invest heavily in tangible items that improve the client experience. At the same time, you may still feel like your business is a disorganized mess on the backend. When the backend of your operations is formal and organized, your experience is improved. You are able to better explain what you do, set reasonable expectations and actually focus on solving a problem for the clients you serve.

This book is important for any practitioner wanting to start or improve their massage practice. Many owners fail in this space because they believe the only important component for having a successful service business is the service itself. We hear it constantly. If the service or product is good, the clients will come. Unfortunately, this way of thinking is flawed.

It is very true that positive reviews and referrals influence new clients to give your business a try. Great service also leads to customers coming back time and time again. However, where many business owners fail, especially in the personal service space, is consistency. This is very likely due to the owner failing to create standard operating procedures. Without a formal standard of operations, owners are leaving everything up to their discretion. This includes things like responding to inquiries, client follow up, service standards, cleanliness, operating hours and more!

Discretion is damaging because it can change on any

given day. Clients prefer a business that is predictable. Predictable does not equal cookie cutter. Clients want to be confident that every time they give you their time and money they will receive the same level of service they fell in love with from day one. As an owner, it is your responsibility to deliver that level of service to every client every time.

It's not just the clients who benefit from formal operations. Owners and staff do as well. Without structure, you are exhausted because you need to figure things out as you go. Nothing becomes ingrained in your business. This makes it difficult to hire and expand your business because your team is never trained to your standards. While they are free to deliver a custom and personalized massage service, they need to know how your business treats the client. There should be no confusion about how to treat the client, what their responsibilities are and what your expectations are. This also takes the power of discretion away from your employees. How confusing would it be if everyone working for you ran your business any way they want.

Leaving the discretion up to employees is too risky. Every one has their own idea of how a business should run, when to do a task and how to perform it. You created your business because you believe your way is the best. Do not allow your staff or yourself to stray from your values, standards or operating procedures.

The breakdown in consistency occurs because the owner has not taken time to formalize these standards. It is my belief that this is neglected because of three reasons. Owners don't find this step to be valuable, they assume everyone intrinsically operates on the same standards, or it feels overwhelming.

This is not a book about how to grow your massage practice, but instead, how to build a strong business with a formal standard operating system in place. You will learn how to create a massage business around the high standards you believe makes you different or even better than all other places. You will also learn how to attract, train and retain a team who values those same standards. Finally, you will learn how to measure and analyze relevant key performance metrics and indicators in the massage industry and what actions to take if they fall below your set benchmarks.

Let's get started!

Kamillya Hunter

1 YOUR IDEAL CLIENT

The idea that delivering an exceptional treatment in the room is all you need to have a successful practice is misleading at best. While there is truth in the statement, it neglects the fact that one must find the right client for their business in the first place not only give an exceptional treatment, but do so consistently. Finding the right client is critical because therapists are able to better explain what it is they do, set reasonable expectations, and actually focus on solving a problem for their client instead of the money.

Have you ever wondered why it is that some massage therapists are able to fill their practice effortlessly with repeat, loyal clients? Have you ever wondered why it is that some places are able to charge double or triple your rates while you find yourself discounting for life? If you are struggling to find your ideal client or build up a loyal client base, there are three things you should do before investing another minute or dollar on your business.

1. Identify the problem you want to solve
2. Understand the solution you provide
3. Have an amazing offer

These things should be done before you begin throwing money at websites and print materials. Before you spend hours recording videos and planning social media content. This should be done before anything else!

Unfortunately, most people completely skip this and end up scrambling to find clients wherever they can. When they fail to connect with the potential clients they do find, they resort to desperate measures like extreme discounting just to get anyone on the table. When you allow pricing to dictate the clients you drive to your practice, you miss out on the clients who are searching for the solution you provide. You leave money on the table.

Pricing is not the only factor that goes into a client's decision to get a massage. More often, they have other reasons for wanting or needing a massage that never seem to be addressed. Too many massage businesses are competing on price instead of expertise. This causes businesses to race to the bottom instead of establishing themselves as the go-to and charging based on the value of their service.

When you don't know what problem you solve, can't articulate your solution, and don't have an offer, it's impossible to begin the discussion of value or worth. So, let's go over those three things you should do before we move any further.

Identify The Problem You Want To Solve

Every person coming for a massage has a problem they

want resolved. Because massage therapists are trained to treat a number of different ailments, there is a tendency to market broadly to capture any and all persons in need of a massage. There is a major problem with that approach.

I've noticed that most massage businesses only focus on pain and/or stress relief. Pain and stress presents itself in many ways. Potential clients find relief in different ways. So while you may offer a solution for chronic pain and stress, so do many other massage therapists and non-massage related services and products. Your solution is only one of many they have to choose from. If you don't know why people choose your service to begin with, you'll have a hard time finding more clients in the future.

I mentioned that pain and stress presents itself to clients in different ways. If that is a problem you can confidently solve, you want to understand every aspect of it. What type of pain do you treat? How long have they been experiencing this pain? How does a client communicate or express that they have this problem? Where do they go to research their problem or search for solutions? Who are the other experts that solve this problem? What type of solutions has the client tried prior to finding you? Once you understand the problem, the key is to speak to *their* language when addressing it.

All over the world there are businesses and clients. Businesses should be obsessed with building awareness and letting people know what it is that they solve, not just what they do. This is because clients are obsessed with finding a solution to a problem that they have, not what a business does. There is a difference.

The business and the client are speaking two different languages. The business is shouting, "Look at our services.

We do all these amazing things. We are the best!" The client is shouting, "I have a problem. Here's how it affects me. Someone please fix it." The businesses that *get it* are the ones who have adjusted their language to one spoken by the client.

The reality is the client does not care how amazing your services are. They don't care about the fancy jargon or credentials. All of that is meaningless if the client doesn't understand how those things work together to solve their problem. That's why it's critical to understand the problem that you solve on a deeper level. Some therapists struggle to identify the problem they solve simply because they are so used to speaking a language very different from a client. They can't hear when a potential client is begging for their services.

It is your responsibility to create a bridge between yourself and the client. It's much easier for the business to adjust their language to attract the clients who are plagued with a specific problem. While this sounds like common sense, many businesses still have not mastered what it means to speak the language of their client once they understand the problem.

Identifying "real problems" can be challenging, but not impossible. Here's an example from a conversation I had with a financial advisor who was struggling to find the language of the market he was trying to reach.

A little over a year ago, a financial advisor was referred to me for content and copywriting services. Having never worked with a financial advisor, I will admit I was a bit nervous before the call. My concern was that I might not be knowledgeable enough about finance to be a good fit. However, the referring party strongly suggested that I hear him out. She was convinced that I could help solve his problem of connecting with his target audience.

During our first call, I asked him a very basic question. How does your service help your client? He spent twenty minutes of the call defining complicated financial terms, explaining how and where he invests their money, and his past experience in working with larger corporate firms. Only he no longer wanted to work with high-income clientele. He wanted to start a business helping lower-income families manage and invest their money. He was not attracting the clients he was seeking.

After five minutes, I could already recognize his problem. He could not communicate effectively with his desired client base because he was still speaking on a corporate level. Many of the clients he was seeking had blue-collar jobs. They didn't want to discuss complicated financial jargon. He thought the jargon impressed that ideal client and made him appear more knowledgeable. The reality is he failed to make the connection.

The clients were not looking to be given a college crash course on high-level finance. These are people who were searching for financial advisors because they had no savings and didn't want to end up working well after 70 like their grandparents. These are people who were scared because they weren't sure how they would pay for their children's college tuition. These people were living check to check and couldn't see how they could even afford to hire a financial advisor AND invest or save for their future. The financial advisor could not connect with them because he was focusing on what he does and how he does it, instead of bridging the gap between their problem and his solution.

The financial advisor needed to listen to his ideal client base. How did they communicate that they were in financial trouble? He needed to weave their language into his and remove all technical jargon. Instead, use theirs. By speaking to his ideal client from their perspective instead of his own, he was able to attract the clientele he was after and fill his courses and client book successfully.

You see, in this example, the financial advisor was able to identify the real problems his ideal clients were dealing with. Their problem wasn't that they simply needed someone to manage their money. It was deeper than that. This is an example of identifying a problem you can and want to solve. Once you have identified the problem, you now need to understand the solution you provide.

Understand The Solution You Provide

There is always more than one solution to a problem. Massage consumers can choose to solve their pain problem with medication, exercise, rest, meditation, massage or any number of options. Of those consumers who choose massage as a desired solution, there are even more options. Luxury spa, franchise, private practice, medical facility, gym, and even in home massage. That still is not an exhaustive list of places they can go for a pain relieving massage.

Even within a single location, clients have their option of different services to achieve their desired health goals. Some clients prefer relaxation to resolve their pain. Others prefer a more aggressive approach. This is why identifying the problem is so critical. Once you've identified the problem, you can begin focusing on a solution.

As massage therapists gain more experience, they begin to specialize in specific modalities. At the very least they have a bit more clarity around the type of services they prefer to provide. A therapist who is trained in oncology massage may want to focus on solving problems unique to cancer patients and survivors. A therapist who is trained in geriatric massage would obviously focus their solutions on that demographic.

This is not to say therapists should only choose one modality or specialty and not diversify. However, one would not use the same language or marketing approach to attract geriatric patients as they would those dealing with cancer. Their problems are not synonymous. While these clients may be in search for the cure for cancer or aging (aren't we all), chances are that's not why they ended up on your massage table. Unless you are confident that you can cure cancer or stop one from aging, it is not enough to just say you provide those types of massage. Especially if the client base is not well informed enough about how that type of service can help them. Your solution must speak to a specific problem each client base faces. Simply having the skill and knowledge alone is not enough. If you are not confident that your solution can solve a problem, do not address it.

I will continue this point with the financial advisor example that was discussed in the previous section.

The financial advisor felt confident that he could solve the three problems he identified within his desired market of clients. To refresh, those problems were: they wanted to be able to retire before age 70, they wanted to be able to afford their children's college tuition and they wanted to know HOW they could afford to hire him, save and invest on a fixed income. Unless he was confident in his solution, he would not address that problem.

His first solution was to teach a basic money management course. Before any client could retain his services, he wanted them to understand basic financial terms, identify areas of wasteful spending and set reasonable and measurable goals they wanted to achieve. This addressed the problem of HOW they could afford to hire him, save and invest even if they were on a fixed income.

The second problem he addressed was retirement goals. Using the information the clients provided in the basic money management course, he would work with them one on one and create an investment strategy depending on their age, desired level of risk and overall retirement goals.

The third problem he addressed was college tuition. Again, using the information obtained during the course, he would work with clients to find the optimal education savings and investment plan based on the age of their child, their future goals and desired level of risk.

As you can probably guess, these solutions are not unique to this one financial advisor. In fact, many advisors provide the same type of service for their clients. On the other hand, the clients could also solve these problems without the assistance of a financial advisor. However, this financial advisor differentiated himself by making the basic money management course a requirement. Educating that demographic was just as important to him as helping them achieve their desired financial goals. He wanted them to know he cared about their financial future and by educating themselves, they could either continue with his services or at the very least, be more informed with whatever method they chose to move forward with.

Understand the solution you have for a specific problem so you can better articulate how you help your client. Then, attract them with an amazing offer.

Have An Amazing Offer

When people hear "amazing offer" it's reasonable to assume price is the focus. Consumers have been conditioned to connect the word offer with discount. Keep in mind, price is not the only reason consumers try new businesses. Yes, many of the larger massage businesses have a low cost introductory offer. That offer is usually cheaper than the normal or membership price to lure new clients in the door. This is not feasible for a lot of smaller massage businesses that lack the brand awareness or staff to handle a high influx of clients at a low price.

An amazing "low price" offer is only one option you could choose. Your offer might be a complimentary gait assessment, complimentary access to spa amenities, extended time, early morning or evening hours, onsite childcare, or a never-ending list of things that are relevant to the problem you are solving for your client.

The offer you present to your clients needs to attract your ideal client. A broad, price-centric offer does nothing to weed out the clients who you cannot or prefer not to help. If your practice focuses on helping athletes minimize recovery time post-event, you might offer a complimentary upgrade to your fire and ice service. You may even consider adding a 15-minute stretch after their session. There is also the option of providing a complimentary welcome gift bag with sports related products from local businesses and products. As you can see the options are limited to the range of your imagination. Relevant and amazing offers will attract the right clients to your door.

To wrap up the example with the financial advisor, I'll share his amazing offer. The market he was trying to reach did not have a lot of disposable income. His offer had to be low enough to be attainable for his ideal clients, but high enough to deter those who were not serious about investing in their financial future. He decided to offer his basic money management course for $99.

The offer was price centric because it would weed out the higher tiered clients that he'd been attracting in the past. His marketing before was all focused on education and high-level financial jargon. The level at which he spoke always attracted white collar six-figure plus clientele. The low cost offer deterred the high level clientele because they assumed the course and services would not be as valuable. The cost as well as the name of the course, basic money management, was not attractive to those who already knew the basics. They wanted the next level. They wanted someone to do these things for them, not learn how to do it themselves. This was key for the financial advisor who wanted to shift his focus to help those who needed it the most.

Unique Selling Point

Now that you have successfully identified the real problems that plague clients as it relates to massage, you can begin to see how it all comes together to form your unique selling point. Your unique selling point is what makes you different from all other massage businesses around. Owners who are clear on their unique selling point have an easier time explaining what they do and why they are better than the competition.

One problem is that many owners base their unique selling point on the small amenities that they offer. Offering aromatherapy, hot towels and heated tables are not unique selling points. These offerings have become the norm within the spa and massage industry. In fact, a client would be more surprised if you didn't offer these amenities than discovering that you do.

Another problem many owners run into is they assume great service is enough to drive clients through the door. Great service might be enough to keep clients, but it is not enough to drive clients. It is certainly not a unique selling point. All businesses believe they have great service. All businesses believe their service is the best, and they should. But not all businesses know what makes them different from a competitor that's two blocks over.

Here is an example. You've identified a major problem in your area. None of the massage businesses in your area offer convenient hours. They all close at 6pm and none are open on Sundays. Your solution is to offer later hours for working adults. A massage business down the street notices the same problem and decides to offer Sunday hours. A third massage business recognizes the same problem and decides to offer in-home services.

As you can see, there is more than one solution to a problem. The actual service of massage is the same, but each business addresses the problem in a different way. Depending on the actual or perceived success of your solution, it is possible that other businesses will follow your lead. The solution will no longer be unique to your business because they will add those solutions as well. This is why innovation and staying on top of trends is so crucial.

This is not to suggest you should chase trends and change your business every time something new comes along. But be aware of the problems that exist and be prepared adjust your business practices if necessary.

Bringing It All Together

Before you can truly find the right clients, you must understand exactly what problem they have, how you solve it, and create an offer that attracts them like magnets. Without clarity on those three places, you will find yourself searching aimlessly for anyone who is willing to come across your table. Sadly, many therapists then rely heavily on those clients to refer to their friends and family. That leads to growth at a snail's pace and is usually not fast enough to sustain the business they are trying to build.

Throughout this book, you will be able to work through many of the topics covered. This will allow you put the information you obtain immediately to use.

With the space provided on the next few pages, break down your client's problem, your solution and the offer you believe will attract them to you. Remember, your business can solve more than one problem. Just make sure you have a specific solution and offer for each problem you solve.

Identify A Real Problem

Understand Your Solution

Your Amazing Offer

2 STANDARDS AND POLICIES

When you run a business where you are the sole owner and operator, you may feel as though creating a formal set of operations is a waste of time. I get it. There are a million other tasks that need to be done. As sole proprietor, you already know how to give a great massage. After all, you attended school and passed your licensing or certification requirements. You may have even gained many years of experience working as a massage therapist from one or more businesses that offer massage treatments. You may have even snagged a few fancy advanced modalities, too.

However, your school teaches you the basic technical skills of performing a massage. When you work for an employer, you are responsible for delivering a service their way. If your employer trained you properly when you were brought on staff, you would have learned about the company history, their standards and policies, your responsibilities, the expectations the company has of you, your expectations of the company, and how your performance would be measured.

Many businesses in this space limit "training" to a tour of the space. They show you where your supplies are, where you will be working, introduce you to coworkers and let you begin immediately. After all, you KNOW how to give a massage and that's what you were hired to do. What more could possible need to be discussed?

Unfortunately, this lack of training is what leads to high employee turnover, disappointment and confusion for everyone involved. My belief is that it's due to owners not dedicating enough time to creating a formal set of operations, standards or policies to support them.

Where should an owner begin?

An owner should begin with their why? Why are you starting your own massage business? When you answer this question honestly, you begin to see where your priorities lie.

There is no right or wrong answer to this question. Many people start businesses, even in the health and wellness space, simply to make money. Others start because they see a need and want to fill it. If you review the introduction chapter, I listed a few of the answers given in the Massage and Spa Business Details That Matter Facebook group.

This is not the time to compare your answer with others, but to reflect on your real reasons for why you want to start your massage business. Using the space below, list all the reasons you want to start your massage business.

Don't worry. This is not a busy task. It is necessary. We will use your responses to identify standards that are important to you. We will then use those standards to build a system to deliver your services efficiently without sacrificing quality. Finally we will create policies to ensure your standards are upheld through service.

I want to start my massage business because…

____

____

____

____

____

____

____

____

____

____

____

____

____

____

____

Standards vs Policies

Let's begin by understanding the difference between standards and policies as it relates to your massage business.

Standard: the level of quality that is used as a measure or model of performance. Standards help set client and employee expectations. Some standards can become part of your unique selling point as well.

Policy: a specific set of rules and guidelines to help establish boundaries for acceptable behavior. From this definition, we can see that policies help support business standards. Policies also contribute to the culture of your company because it helps to enforce expectations to both clients and employees.

Your business standards and policies should be consistent and support one another. Here is an example of consistent standards and policies within a massage practice:

Every Touch Massage (ETM) promises that clients will be greeted with fresh steeped tea prior to their session, have a warm table waiting for them when it's time to begin their session, and receive a custom massage treatment that focuses on their needs that day. These are basic standards of service that ETM has instilled in their business.

To ensure these standards are upheld, ETM has policies in place for BOTH the clients and staff. ETM recommends that clients arrive at least 15 minutes prior to the start of their appointment time. This allows them to select their choice of tea and enjoy the beverage without feeling rushed.

ETM also requires that massage therapists arrive at least 15 minutes prior to the start of their service so they can prepare the room, warm the table, and review the clients intake form or pre-session interview. The massage therapist is expected to do an intake with every client every time, even if the client is a regular. Because one of the standards is that clients will receive a custom massage session that focuses on their needs *that day*, this is a critical policy that ensures the client is satisfied with their most recent visit.

Without those types of policies in place to support those standards, clients may not understand why they didn't receive fresh tea if they arrived immediately at the start of their appointment time. If there is no policy in place for the massage therapist to arrive 15 minutes early for their session, the promise of the table being warm may not be kept. Understandably, it may not take 15 minutes for a massage table to heat to a warm and comfortable temperature. The 15 minutes is also to make sure the therapist is not rushing. They have time to set up their room, check their schedule for the day, use the restroom, or simply relax before it's time for their workday to begin.

The example used is very basic. It does not go into the specific operating protocols, but highlights just a few standards and policies that a business might have in place. We will dive further into creating operating procedures around those standards and policies in the next segment.

For now, let's review the answers you gave in the previous section. You were asked to list the reasons why you started your own massage business. Looking over those answers, how many of them had to do with the client's experience? How many had to do with your experience as an employee? Separate those answers into two different groups.

Examples of reasons surrounding client experience would be:

- I didn't like that I had to rush through sessions
- We didn't keep proper SOAP notes or client records
- Clients would no show or cancel at the last minute without consequence
- Clients would be double booked
- Lack of cleanliness

Examples surrounding your experience as an employee would be:

- I was overbooked
- I always felt rushed
- There was no opportunity for career advancement
- I needed freedom and flexibility with my schedule
- I felt undervalued, unappreciated, and underpaid
- I wanted more control
- I CAN'T work for someone else

Whatever reasons you listed speak to some of the things

you value most. The goal is to take those values and create a set of standards. These standards will be the building blocks for how your business will treat both clients and employees. Even if you do not have employees or never intend to have any, the standards apply to you as well. After all, you deserve to be treated well, too.

It is the owner's responsibility to determine the standards, create the policies and set an example for how everyone should be treated and behave. As the owner and operator, it's even more critical for you to respect and uphold the standards you set. Clients should always feel like they will consistently receive a great service, even if you are the only person available to deliver them.

Using just a few of the examples listed above, here are a few standards and policies you can create based on those reasons:

Client Experience:

- *I didn't like that I had to rush through sessions*

  Standard: Services a full 60 or 90 minute sessions. Therapists will have 15 minutes between scheduled sessions to account for thorough client intake, room change over, and post session follow-up.

  Policies: Clients need to arrive at least 5 minutes prior to appointment time to ensure they receive maximum time on the table. Therapists greet their client on time. The 15-minute buffer between clients is not meant to be extra hands-on massage time. The massage sessions will be a full 60 or 90 minutes of hands on time with the remaining time being dedicated to intake, cleaning, and follow-up.

- *We didn't keep proper SOAP notes or client records*

  Standard: We will keep SOAP notes and client records up to date at all times.

  Policy: Clients must provide accurate information at every visit. Staff must update notes prior to leaving for the day.

Employee Experience:

- *I was overbooked*

  Standard: Therapists will not work beyond their physical capacity. Therapists will be scheduled a full 30 to 60-minute uninterrupted lunch break.

  Policy: Therapist must inform the scheduling manager of their massage capacity. Changes to massage capacity must be presented two weeks in advance in writing unless due to an emergency or physical injury.

- *I felt undervalued, underappreciated, and underpaid*

Standard: Every employee is valued, appreciated and are fairly compensated.

Policy: Each employee will receive a biannual review where performance and salary will be discussed. Employees will be trained and clearly understand their responsibilities expectations and pay scale prior to beginning work.

To some of you reading, those examples may seem like common sense. To others they may seem outrageous and even unnecessary. Standards and policies vary widely between the many different massage businesses. Think about your own. Some of these may already be implemented, even if they aren't formalized. Some, you may have never considered. An important thing to remember is that you are allowed to determine and improve your standards as your business matures. You are allowed to modify and add new policies as new issues or concerns arise.

Some of your current standards and policies may feel like second nature. This is not the case for everyone. Many owners have no desire to create cancellation policies. Many owners have never considered formalizing a standard for how clients are treated when they walk in the door. That alone confirms that just because YOU have an idea of how clients should be treated does not mean others are required or expected to agree with you. This goes for both employees and clients.

It's the reason so many different massage businesses

exist in the first place. No two are exactly the same. Every owner has a different reason for why they chose to open. Every owner has a different answer for what makes their massage practice different or better than the next. And every client has a different set of expectations and a different opinion of what policies they choose to accept. The same is true for employees. This is why it's so important for owners to know what standards they value and what policies make sense to uphold those standards.

The right standards and policies will help you attract clients who are looking for that level of service. It will retain clients who want to receive that great service consistently. If will attract employees whose standards are in alignment with your own. It will retain employees who understand the importance of their contribution and that the company cares just as much about them as they do the client.

Now you have a better understanding of why standards and policies are so valuable to your business, your clients and your staff. Use the space provided over the next few pages to begin creating some policies and standards based on the answers you listed earlier for why you decided to start your massage business.

The goal is not to create the perfect standards or policies. The goal is to have a foundation that you can build on. For now, we simply want to identify a few points that stand out to you when you consider your ideal business and place of work.

List the reasons you decided to start your business that have to do with the client experience:

____

____

____

____

____

____

____

____

____

____

____

____

____

____

____

____

List the standards that coincide with those reasons:

List the policies that you can put in place to support those standards:

____

____

____

____

____

____

____

____

____

____

____

____

____

____

____

____

List the reasons you decided to start your business that have to do with your experience as an employee:

List the standards that coincide with those answers:

____

____

____

____

____

____

____

____

____

____

____

____

____

____

____

____

List the policies that you can put in place to support those standards:

____

____

____

____

____

____

____

____

____

____

____

____

____

____

____

____

3 THE CLIENT JOURNEY

The client's journey begins long before they step foot into your massage business. It begins the moment they are introduced to your brand. This could happen on social media, through a personal referral, an online search, or a postcard that came in the mail. However they heard about your business is the moment their journey begins. Your goal is to extend that journey as long as possible.

For the purpose of this book, we will only focus on the time they decide to schedule an appointment to the time they pay for their session and leave. Later, I will break this journey down into three important segments for the sake of you creating your operating procedures without feeling overwhelmed with the process.

For now, I will give a brief overview of the client journey and identify some critical touch points along the way. Let's imagine what the journey may feel like from the client's perspective.

The client is introduced to your business by referral. They hear all about your amazing services and can't wait to experience it for themselves. At this point they have made the decision to give you their money.

Scheduling The Appointment

Scheduling the appointment is the first critical touch point. Many clients have a preference in how they would like to schedule their appointments. Some prefer only to speak to someone over the phone. Some are comfortable scheduling themselves online. Some are open to communicating through messenger, email or text. Some take their chances by walking in unannounced.

There is no right or wrong way to schedule an appointment. Only preference. If your company is open to all scheduling options, it is important to make that clear. If you do not accept walk-in appointments, you will likely turn away clients who prefer only to walk in the day of their appointment. If you do not have a receptionist or answering service readily available to answer client calls, you will likely miss out on clients who prefer to speak with someone when scheduling their service.

As the owner, it is up to you to decide how your clients are able to schedule their appointments. While technological advances have made it easier for clients to schedule themselves, remember, clients have their preferences as well. They may not want to create another account, provide their information online, or they may have questions and simply want them answered prior to scheduling. It is okay to only allow scheduling online. It is okay to only allow scheduling over the phone. It is okay to not take walk-in appointments. Just make sure your scheduling procedures are clear and consistent.

Consistency is important because you never know how a new client is introduced to you. If your business has a policy that you do not accept walk-in appointments, but all of your reviews praise you for accepting them the same day they just walked into your practice, it can be confusing. They may not know you only allow existing clients to walk-in. They may not know you only allow referrals to walk-in. Whatever your scheduling practices are, they need to be clear and consistent.

Appointment Confirmation

Now your client has scheduled their appointment. Both parties are excited and looking forward to the service. It is standard practice in this industry to confirm appointments between 72-24 hours prior to the service. You can decide to confirm appointments via text, email or phone. Creating a script or template for how you would like your business to confirm appointments is simple and takes all of the guesswork out of the task. Not all massage businesses confirm their appointments. Those that do, experience a lower percentage of last minute cancellations and no shows.

Check-In

Clients arrive to their appointment with certain expectations. If they have received a massage from your company before, they are expecting to be greeted and treated the same way every time they come back. If this is their first experience at your massage business, they may be basing their expectations on what was told to them via referral, public reviews or experiences they've had at other businesses that are similar to yours. This emphasizes the significance of consistency through formal procedures. You want every client to have an amazing and predictable experience every time.

This can be achieved by communicating policies and expectations prior to them arriving. If the client is new, you may want to share some information with them. When they schedule their appointment or when you do confirmations, let them know how early they should arrive to complete paperwork and relax a bit before the start. If you work alone, let them know if no one is up front to greet them to simply wait quietly until the previous session ends. If you offer optional snacks, drinks or a foot soak prior to the start of their session, mention these luxuries before they arrive to their first appointment so they give themselves enough time to enjoy them all.

If you have improved or changed any of your pre-session offerings, make sure you mention them prior to your client arriving. Clients may be anticipating things you no longer offer. Letting them know about changes prior to their arrival manages their expectations and helps to improve their overall experience.

Meeting The Therapist

If you are a solo owner and operator, you may want to inform new clients of this fact. Many massage businesses have a front desk staff that is fully separate from the massage staff. A new client may assume your practice is set up the same way.

When a client schedules their appointment, it may be benefit everyone to mention that you, the therapist, will be greeting them when they arrive and providing their service. It can be a shock to a client who has never been to a small private practice where the therapist does everything. They may need to mentally prepare for the fact that there will be no buffer between paying, tipping and providing feedback for their experience. If you have a full staff, your therapist will be introduced or may introduce themselves to the client.

Please note, the presence of a full staff or the lack of one does not necessarily attract or deter a client. There can be benefits to each. Some clients like to know they are working directly with the owner. They may like that their money and feedback are heard by the exact person in charge of decision making.

Client Interview

During the client interview, the next critical touch point arises. If your massage practice requires an intake form to be completed, the massage therapist will review it with the client in private, confirm the type of service the client would like to receive, and possibly recommend an upgrade or different service based on their needs. This part is critical because it catches any scheduling errors and misunderstandings. It also gives the client and massage therapist the opportunity to understand and agree on what will happen during the session. Each party can better prepare and adjust their expectations accordingly.

Comfort Checks

The comfort check is another critical and sometimes overlooked touch point. Because comfort is subjective, the therapist is responsible for delivering on this touch point. This can be achieved by simply asking and checking in on things like temperature, music volume, pressure and anything else that can be adjusted. As the owner, you set the standard for how frequently your massage therapists need to check in about comfort.

It is important to note that setting a standard for how to and how frequently your massage therapists perform comfort checks does not impede with their massage. Standardizing comfort checks does not create a cookie cutter service, but makes sure clients are not injured, disappointed, or unimpressed with their service.

Many therapists will agree that they customize their massage to their client's needs. A service cannot be customized to a client's preference or needs if they are never asked about those things to begin with. Comfort and needs can change throughout the session, so only asking at the start may not be enough. Comfort checks are in place to improve the client experience and decrease negative feedback and complaints about the service in the treatment room.

Post-Massage Interview

After the massage is over, many therapists review the session with the client. This is the time to discuss what the therapist felt during the session, get immediate feedback from the client, and make recommendations or referrals for future services. Not all post session follow-ups are that in depth. Depending on the type of massage environment, referrals and future appointment recommendations may not be appropriate, necessary or required.

Obviously there are benefits to a good thorough follow-up. The massage therapist and client are able to give and receive immediate feedback. The therapist can assess the changes in areas such as range of motion, gait and even pain levels. The client is able to ask questions about self-care, address concerns, and even provide direct feedback to the therapist if they feel comfortable doing so.

Check-Out

Once the session is complete, the client needs to check out. This is also the last critical touch point for your client. This could be the last time your business ever has contact with the client. At this time, they may need to pay for their session if they haven't paid in advance. This is also a good time to ask for feedback, schedule the client's next appointment, or attempt to sell a package or membership if applicable.

Now that we've given a brief overview of the client journey, the next upcoming chapters will break down the three important segments of the journey. Before The Session, During The Session and After The Session.

4 CREATING OPERATING PROCEDURES

As we break down our client's journey, we want to take note of all the components that make up each segment. It is you, the owner, who decides what happens at each step. Without standards, policies and procedures, you leave everything up to the discretion of your employees or yourself based on mood. So here is where you will decide what and how everything is done.

Once everyone knows how to perform their given tasks, they need to be performing them consistently. Consistency matters because it helps establish a routine that will eventually become second nature.

As we build on your procedures, keep in mind there is always information you will need to share with the client and information they need to share with you.

I. Before The Session

A lot of things take place before your client receives their massage. As we briefly discussed, a new client can be introduced to your business a number of different ways.

When they decide to schedule their appointment is where we will begin creating your formal operating procedures.

A lot happens before your client arrives for an appointment. First, they need to schedule. Before they can even do that, the client needs to know things like cost, hours of operations, how to schedule, and payment options. You may want to include this information on your marketing collateral, website and social media platforms.

Let's assume you do not have any limitations on how your clients can schedule an appointment with you, so they decide to call. This is where your protocols begin.

RESOURCE: Prior to the session, many massage businesses require that clients complete an intake form. If you do not have one, you can find many at www.mymassageworld.com/free-support/free-forms/

Scheduling An Appointment

How does your company respond to appointment requests? (email, text, phone call, etc?)

____

____

____

How soon does your company respond? (Same day, within 24 hours, etc?)

____

____

____

Who is responsible for responding to appointment requests? (front desk team, automated online scheduler, etc?)

____

____

____

How soon are new clients able to schedule an appointment? (Same day, 48 hours, etc?)

____

____

____

What specific information do you need from new clients? Existing clients? (Name, contact information, service preferences, therapist request, etc?)

____

____

____

What specific information does your client need from you? (Location, directions, recommended arrival time, etc?)

____

____

____

Is there anything that is required before the client can

schedule an appointment? (credit card on file, questionnaire, agree to policies, etc?)

____

____

____

Appointment Confirmations

Do you confirm appointments?

____

____

____

How is this done?

____

____

____

How far in advance?

____

____

____

Who is responsible for this task?

____

____

____

If the appointment is not confirmed, what happens?

____

____

____

Arriving For The Appointment

How soon should a new client arrive for their appointment? Existing client?

____

____

____

How are clients greeted when they arrive?

____

____

____

Who is responsible for greeting the client?

____

____

____

What information do you need from the client when they arrive? (Name, health info, etc)

____

____

____

How is this information collected?

____

____

____

Where is this information stored?

____

____

____

How soon is the information stored?

____

____

____

How long do you keep this information?

____

____

____

Who has access to this information?

____

____

____

What information does the client need from you prior to the start of the session?

What amenities are available to the client prior to the start of their service? (Snacks, beverages, sauna, private waiting area, etc?)

Who is responsible for offering or serving these amenities? (Front desk, therapist, self-serve?)

What happens if the client arrives late for their appointment?

Meeting The Massage Therapist

What time does the client meet the therapist? (5 minutes prior to appointment time, at appointment time, within first 5 minutes, etc?)

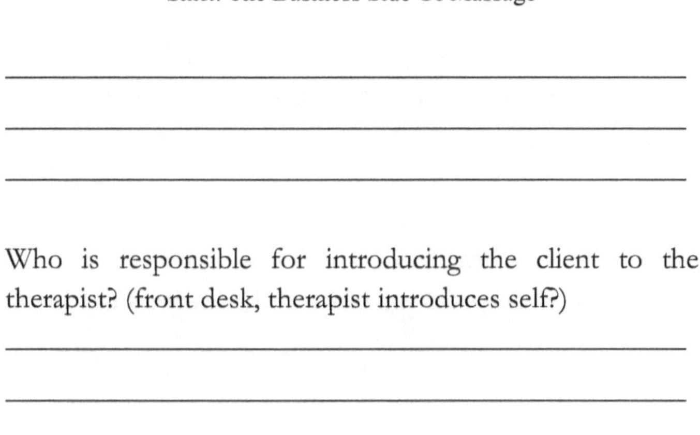

____

____

____

Who is responsible for introducing the client to the therapist? (front desk, therapist introduces self?)

____

____

____

II. During The Session

The entire massage session begins the moment the massage therapist takes the client back to the treatment room. Massage sessions don't just begin. Therapists perform a pre-session interview in the treatment room. This is the opportunity for the therapist to confirm the type of massage, find out if there are any contraindications, and even upgrade the client to a more advanced treatment.

While every massage therapist performs their service in a unique way, as the owner, you still have a say in how the client is treated during the session. Requiring comfort checks, upselling, and set hands-on time removes all discretion from your employees. What stops your massage therapists from cutting your clients short? What stops your massage therapists from assuming they know what is best for the client? The answer is your standards, policies and procedures.

During the session is over after the massage therapist performs the post-session interview. This is a great time for the therapist to review the session, answer questions and possibly encourage the client to schedule future appointments.

Pre-Session Interview

What information does the therapist have access to?

____

____

____

What information does the therapist need from the client?

____

____

____

How long should the pre-session interview last? (2 minutes, 5 minutes, as long as necessary, etc?)

____

____

____

What types of questions should be asked? (Medical history, session preference, upsell/upgrade, etc?)

____

____

____

How does the therapist record and store the information they've collected?

____

____

____

Massage Session

How long does the hands-on session last?

____

____

____

What amenities are required in every session? (Hot towels, aromatherapy, eye pillow, etc?)

____

____

____

How soon should the therapist ask about client comfort?

____

____

____

How often should the therapist ask?

____

____

____

Is there a minimum number of comfort checks that must be met?

____

____

____

What specific comforts should the therapist be concerned with? (Temperature, pressure, music volume, etc?)

____

____

____

How is the massage affected if the client arrives late?

____

____

____

How are these consequences communicated to the client?

____

____

____

Is it ever acceptable for the therapist to give extra massage time?

____

____

____

Post-Massage Interview

What information is asked, shared, and recorded during the interview?

____

____

____

What information MUST be given to the client prior to check out?

____

____

____

How is this information recorded and stored?

____

____

____

Who has access to this information?

____

____

____

How soon should this information be stored?

____

____

____

How long is this information stored?

____

____

____

III. After The Session

After the post-massage interview is complete, the client needs to check out. There may be information or feedback you would like to obtain from your client. You are in this "segment" until the client returns for their next session. There are steps that need to take place when collecting information, payment and even following up with your clients.

You may treat clients who immediately reschedule different from clients who reschedule at a later time. There may be incentives you decide to offer for regular clients versus infrequent ones. This is all up to you, the owner to decide.

Many owners who are sole operators find this to be the most uncomfortable part in the client journey. The potential for negative feedback, the need to sell and schedule future appointments and collect payment can be filled with anxiety. Creating a script and a procedure that includes best practices for checking out your clients helps remove the anxiety.

If you have a front desk staff that is responsible for checking out the clients, they also need scripts and training on how you would like them to collect payment, receive feedback and how to convert clients into members. Without a script or standard you risk leaving things up to your staff's discretion. Do you want them to always ask for client feedback? Do you want them to always recommend that the client reschedule? Do you want them to always attempt to sell your membership (if applicable)?

If your answer is yes to any of these questions, they need to know how you want them to do these tasks. How many attempts should they make? One? Three? Ten? Without knowing they are left deciding for themselves and each client will receive a different experience depending on who checks them out and how they feel that day. We have already established that discretion is not favorable.

In addition to checking out the client, your business also needs to be cleaned. This includes places like the treatment rooms, break room, storage area, restrooms, locker rooms, lobby, hallways, etc. It also includes little things like door knobs, windows, computers, service supplies, trash, dishes, etc. Many owners assume that staff will simply share these responsibilities. That is not the case. The tasks should be distributed as you see fit and all parties need to be aware of their responsibilities and expectations.

Check-Out

Who is responsible for checking out the client?

____

____

____

Who is responsible for collecting payment?

____

____

____

What information is collected prior to the client leaving?

____

____

____

Does the client have access to any amenities prior to leaving?

____

____

____

Will the client be asked to reschedule?

____

____

____

Will the client be asked to join a membership? (If

applicable)

____

____

____

Is there any incentive for clients who reschedule immediately?

____

____

____

Is the client sent home with anything? (Brochures, water, free samples?)

____

____

____

Will the client be receiving any follow up marketing materials? (Email, thank you card, gift voucher, etc?)

____

____

____

Who is responsible for following up with the client?

____

____

____

How soon do you follow up?

____

____

____

How often do you follow up?

____

____

____

Cleaning Duties

How often is your lobby cleaned?

____

____

____

Who is responsible for this task?

____

____

____

How will you ensure this task has been completed?

____

____

____

How often are treatment rooms cleaned (vacuuming, dusting, walls, etc.)? Who is responsible for this task?

____

____

____

How will you ensure this task has been completed?

____

____

____

How often is the hallway cleaned? Who is responsible for this task?

____

____

____

How will you ensure this task has been completed?

____

____

____

How often are the restrooms cleaned (both employee and client)? Who is responsible for this task?

____

____

____

How will you ensure this task has been completed?

____

____

____

How often is the break room cleaned? Who is responsible for this task?

____

____

____

How will you ensure this task has been completed?

____

____

____

How often is the storage area cleaned? Who is responsible for this task?

____

____

____

How will you ensure this task has been completed?

____

____

____

How often does your practice get deep cleaned? (door knobs, keyboards, office supplies and equipment, treatment supplies and equipment, phones, etc) Who is responsible for this task?

____

____

____

How often is laundry done? Who is responsible for this task?

____

____

How will you ensure this task has been completed?

____

____

____

IV. Bonus Segment: Memberships

Memberships are an amazing way to generate recurring revenue within your massage business. There are a number of spa and massage businesses that have implemented a membership in their business model and have experienced great success. If you intend to add a membership to your practice, please review the following questions.

You may not have all the answers. For many of them, you may not know how to resolve it until the situation arises. In the meantime, it is important that you at least give thought to them. It is a strong chance that you and your team will experience all of these questions/issues. If you have read Success Of A Failed Therapist, this next segment is not new to you.

MEMBERSHIP BASICS

How much is your membership?

____

____

____

Are there different levels to your membership?

____

____

____

What does your membership include?

____

____

____

What additional privileges or incentives do members have over non-members?

____

____

____

Does the membership just include a massage?

____

____

____

What length of massage does one get with the membership?

____

____

____

Does this include add-ons (aromatherapy, hot stones, etc)?

____

____

____

What about advanced services (prenatal, sports, deep tissue, etc)?

____

____

____

TERMS

Do clients have to sign a contract? (clients ask this all the time)

____

____

____

Is there a fee to cancel?

____

____

____

Is there a rescission period?

____

____

Are clients "locked in"?

____

____

____

How can clients cancel? (in person only, in writing, through email, verbally, etc)

____

____

____

Do clients need to give notice? (2 weeks, 1 month, 3 months, etc)

____

____

____

What if your client moves?

____

____

____

What if the client can't afford the payments?

____

____

____

Can a client put their membership on hold?If so, how long?

____

____

____

Can clients upgrade their membership?

____

____

____

Can clients downgrade their membership?

____

____

____

How often can a client switch between memberships?

____

____

____

THOSE TRICKY PAYMENT ISSUES

When will membership payment be drafted?

____

Can clients choose their draft date?

If the payment fails, will you attempt to retry?

If so, how soon will you attempt to retry the payment?

Will you notify the client if you attempt to retry the payment?

How will you notify a client of a retry attempt?

How will you notify a client that their payment failed?

How many times will you attempt to retry the payment if it fails?

Are clients penalized or charged a fee for failed payments?

Is the membership still active after a failed payment?

Will you cancel a membership after a failed payment?

How do clients notify you if they change their bank information?

____

____

____

How soon before the draft date do clients need to notify you of new banking information?

____

____

____

THOSE DANG UNUSED SESSIONS

Do unused sessions roll over?

____

____

____

Can someone else use the prepaid session?

____

____

____

Is there a fee to allow someone else to use prepaid sessions?

____

____

____

How many people are allowed to use the prepaid sessions?

____

____

____

How many times can clients add or change who is allowed to use the membership?

____

____

____

Can clients convert their sessions into gift certificates?

____

____

____

Is there a fee to convert the sessions into gift certificates?

____

____

____

Can clients get a refund on unused sessions? (check your local laws before you decide)

____

____

____

Do you set a limit on unused sessions?

____

____

____

If so, will the client's membership be cancelled when that limit is reached?

____

____

____

Will you notify clients of unused sessions?

____

____

____

How soon will you begin notifying clients of unused sessions? How often

____

____

____

THOSE UNCOMFORTABLE POLICIES

If a client last minute cancels or no shows, is their prepaid session charged?

____

If a client last minute cancels or no shows, are they charged the membership price or non-member rate?

What happens if the person using a client's sessions last minute cancels or no-shows?

Is the client's card charged or is their pre-paid session charged?

If the client knows the money won't be in their account on the draft date, are they allowed to request a later date?

How many times can a client change their draft date?

____

____

____

Do you allow clients to "gift" memberships?

____

____

____

If the recipient of a "gifted" membership last minute cancels or no shows, who is charged?

____

____

____

Who is allowed to cancel the membership? (spouse, friend, parent, child, caretaker)

____

____

____

OH CRAP! WE SCREWED UP!

What happens if you overcharged a client's account?

____

____

____

What happens if you draft on the wrong date?

____

____

____

What happens if you've over drafted a client's account and caused them fees?

____

____

____

The client cancelled and you still charged them. How soon can they expect a refund?

____

____

____

What if a client is unhappy with the services?

____

____

____

THE UNTHINKABLE

A client only signed up for a specific therapist. That therapist quit. Can they cancel?

____

____

The client is moving. Can they cancel without penalty?

____

____

____

A doctor says your client can't get a massage anymore. Can they cancel without penalty?

____

____

____

A client was injured. Can they cancel without penalty?

____

____

____

Wrapping Up

Hopefully you were able to answer all the questions regarding your client experience. This is how your formal operating procedures begin to take shape. If and when complaints and inefficiencies arise, you are better able to identify what went wrong and how you can improve your procedures or policies to manage against them.

Again, this is not meant to be set in stone, but to give you a basic starting point from which you can add or modify as you put them in action and train yourself and staff to them.

I recognize this is not an all encompassing list. Use the space available on the next few pages to add any steps that may be missing or are critical to how your massage business operates.

5 RECRUITING, TRAINING, AND RETAINING YOUR TEAM

Hopefully you have spent a significant amount of time working through the details of how your business operates. Whether you are working your business solo or plan to have employees, the best thing you can do for everyone involved is have a formal standard of operating procedures. Your clients will appreciate the consistency. You will feel less overwhelmed with the tasks. Your staff will actually know what their job entails and how they are supposed to do it.

According to numerous industry resources, one of the reasons for such high turnover in the massage and spa industry is lack of training and poor support from management. If you have ever worked as an employee in the industry, you might agree that it is very high on the reasons for why massage therapists quit. Pay is not always the leading factor.

In fact, many massage therapists stated the reason they

quit in regards to pay is because they were required to do more tasks than just massage. They felt their wage did not reflect the amount of work they were expected to do. Problems like this are avoided when owners formally outline the operating procedures, properly delegate each task, train the staff on how to perform the task, clearly communicate the responsibilities and expectations, and provide feedback on performance.

In the previous section, you should have outlined your operating procedures and listed who would be responsible for each task. Review your procedures and who is responsible. Does anything appear unbalanced? Imagine if you were responsible for the tasks you listed. What type of salary do you think would be sufficient? (Pro Tip: If you are not sure what salary should align with that position, search local job offerings. Avoid asking social media groups that are not local to you. Each state has different minimum wage requirements and average cost of living. For example, California's cost of living is much higher than Ohio. A receptionist might willingly accept $10 an hour in Ohio, but maybe not in California.)

A close second to overworked and underpaid, is lack of benefits. There are countless benefits massage business owners can provide to their employees. Many states and professional associations require massage therapists to obtain continuing educations credits either annually or biannually. Employers who provide or offer to pay for continuing education courses are attractive to therapists who are looking for more than just a salary.

Other benefits that attract massage therapists are opportunities for career advancement, flexibility in scheduling, control over the type of massage they provide, the ability to work in the same position without restrictions, the ability to pursue their own business interests, mentorship and connections with seasoned therapists, paid time off, health insurance, retirement plans and much more.

The reality is, if pay and benefits were enough to keep a good employee, no one would ever quit their jobs if those two concerns were met. Unfortunately we know this is not the case.

Earlier in the book, you were asked to list the reasons you chose to start your own massage business. Did you even mention health insurance, the fact that continuing education courses weren't covered, or lack of mentorship? Probably not. You may be one of many who listed a reason that had to do with a poor work experience. The same reason many massage therapists start their own business is also the same reason many of them quit their jobs and search for a new one. Many therapists are searching for better opportunities whether they like their current employer or not.

Recruiting

According to the American Massage Therapy Association, there are over 300,000 massage therapists in the United States. Yet one of the biggest complaints of employers is a lack of qualified candidates. Students are graduating from school with poor table side manners, lack of hands on experience and confidence, or simply poor work ethic.

If you are currently an employee, and have never had the responsibility of hiring a massage staff, this may be news to you. However, this is a concern that arises all over the country. Though massage therapists have their reasons for quitting, employers have valid reasons for terminating or never offering employment. Tardiness, constant call offs, poor customer service, refusal to perform tasks in the manner they were trained and many other concerns make finding reliable and responsible employees a challenging effort.

As an employer, it is your responsibility to recruit a team that aligns with your values, standards and possesses the qualities and qualifications your company requires. The same energy must be applied to attracting your ideal staff as you do your ideal client. After all, they are the ones who will be delivering your amazing services to those clients. When those clients are treated poorly, it makes the business look bad. So how do you find those team members who would be a perfect fit?

Begin by identifying the type employees you will need. Typically in a smaller practice you will at least need a massage therapist and a receptionist. Someone should be responsible for things like general office tasks like answering phones, filing paperwork, storing client information, greeting and checking out clients, etc. Someone needs to be responsible for performing the service, maintaining cleanliness, ordering supplies, stocking supplies, and so on. If you plan to be an absent owner, you may also want to hire a manager. Their responsibilities may include interviewing and hiring new staff, training, HR, payroll, managing KPIs, customer service, etc.

Once you have identified the type of employees you need, be specific about what their responsibilities will be. The more specific and clear, the better. This doesn't mean that other employees can not help out with tasks that are outside their job description. But this comes back to removing discretion. If you do not identify what someone's responsibilities are, you leave it up to their discretion. Your expectations may differ from theirs in regards to basic tasks that need to be performed and who should complete them.

An example would be laundry. If you do not hire an outside entity to perform laundry services, someone needs to perform this task. Is it the responsibility of the massage therapists? If the massage therapists are busy and have no time to wash, dry, fold and stock linens, will the front desk be expected to perform these tasks? Questions like this come up frequently in massage businesses. It is the owner's responsibility to delegate tasks and give specific guidelines for how they should be performed.

Using your operations outline from the previous chapter, what staff members do you need for your business to operate?

____

____

____

____

____

____

____

____

Even if you plan to actively work in your business, don't leave your responsibilities out. Remember, you are building a business that eventually will be able to function with or without your presence.

Now that you have identified your core staff, you will need to list the responsibilities of each of them. Again, try to be as specific as possible when detailing the tasks that will be performed. Some tasks, like in the laundry example, may be shared. Other tasks, such as handling money or clients information, may require exclusivity.

You may find that the business you are trying to open requires more than just 3 types of employees (massage therapist, receptionist, manager). If you plan to open a full service spa, you may also need estheticians, manicurist, cosmetologists, cleaning staff, leads, or more. Depending on your business size and goals, use the space below to identify the positions you need and what their specific responsibilities will be.

You may not have all the answers now, but this is a great place to start. You will use this information to determine things like salary, bonuses, benefits, etc. If you are not sure where to start, try searching local listings for the positions you identified to get an idea of what other businesses list in their job descriptions. Compare that to the outline of your operations that you created in the previous chapter.

You may disagree with the responsibilities other businesses require of their employees. That is okay. The goal is to eventually create a job posting that will attract your ideal staff. Staff members who feel the pay is not compatible with the responsibilities will not want to work for you. Those who agree will express their interest.

Employee Title and Responsibilities:

____

____

____

____

____

____

____

____

____

____

____

Employee Title and Responsibilities:

____

____

____

____

____

____

____

____

____

____

____

____

Employee Title and Responsibilities:

____

____

____

____

____

____

____

____

____

____

Employee Title and Responsibilities:

____

____

____

____

____

____

____

____

____

____

____

Now that you have outlined the title and basic responsibilities of your future (or current) team, you can begin assigning a salary to the position. Remember, salary is only one component. Many employees are attracted to other benefits that are not offered everywhere.

If you happen to be an employer who offers any of the benefits discussed earlier, you'll want to advertise them. Finding an employer who offers any of the benefits listed above is challenging. It is not something most massage therapists expect because it is so rare to find. A lot of seasoned therapists gravitate to businesses that are thoughtful and stable enough to provide benefits.

If your massage business is more established and you have already or are in the process of hiring a receptionist, the same principles apply. Even receptionists look for advancement, training opportunities and benefits.

They may not recognize or appreciate the importance of their position within a massage business, but it is your job to help them get there. A good receptionist provides customer service, scheduling and organization. A great receptionist excels at conflict resolution, understands the different benefits of massage to guide the client to the right service, and upsells to drive more revenue into the business. A great receptionist knows their value and likely has experience in the position.

It is not necessary to only recruit experienced employees. While that does help with the learning curve, you may suffer when it comes to the training curve. Their experience, while extremely valuable, could conflict with the way you do business. Avoid relying on experience and search for signs of trainability.

Regardless of how much experience a new employee has, they still need to be trained to your business procedures. This ensures they are performing tasks consistently to your standards. Your clients chose your business for a reason. It is important that your staff understands this. If they do not agree with how you do things, there are two options: start their own business or find another employer who they are more compatible with. This is not to suggest that everything is either your way or the highway. There should be an understanding that they at least need to respect how you do things.

However, their experience should not be ignored. They may have valuable tips and suggestions regarding efficiency, sales and service tips. Listen to your staff, both new and existing because their recommendations and feedback could make the difference in providing your clients with good service or amazing service.

Use this space provided to identify the salary your will offer and the qualifications you desire of your team. If you cannot afford to pay your staff competitive wages or benefits, you may only end up attracting candidates with less experience. Hope is not lost. There are great candidates out there who lack experience. There are also great candidates with tons of experience who are not driven by salary. The goal is to be clear about your qualifications such as years of experience, values, training, etc. The expectations and requirements you provide will hopefully weed out the unqualified people.

Employee Title, Salary and Requirements:

____

____

____

____

____

____

____

____

____

____

____

Employee Title, Salary and Requirements:

____

____

____

____

____

____

____

____

____

____

Employee Title, Salary and Requirements:

____

____

____

____

____

____

____

____

____

____

____

____

Employee Title, Salary and Requirements:

____

____

____

____

____

____

____

____

____

____

You now have a good idea of who you need, what you want to pay, and the qualifications you are looking for. Very soon you will discover that finding the right staff can me just as challenging and expensive as finding the right client.

Just as you would market and advertise your business to attract clients, the same applies to staff. There are many places to search for qualified staff. Some owners recruit students right out of school. Others pay for ads on job sites like indeed.com or salonjobs.com. You can also announce your openings via social media, professional associations or wherever massage therapists are likely to be present.

If you are having trouble deciding where to start advertising your job opening, begin by contacting local schools in your area. Many schools offer job placement services that benefit both the students and local businesses in the area. It is possible they will post your opening, send an email or even host a job fair to help get former students placed.

Another place to start is by searching for the job you are advertising yourself. A quick internet search will yield many results. You will find out how and where other businesses are advertising their openings and you can do the same.

If you already have staff, do not overlook them as a resource for recruiting other staff members. It is very likely that if they are happy with their place of employment, they will want their friends to work there as well.

Your website can act as a good place to recruit staff as well. Generally, massage therapists and other candidates who are searching for employment will search in their area.

Many of them will inquire directly with the business about job openings either through email or phone call. Some may even just pop up and ask in person. If you have a preference for how you want candidates to apply, make sure it is clear on your website and your existing staff are knowledgeable about how to handle those inquiries. You may not be actively recruiting, but it is much better to have a bank of resumes and applications to choose from than to search out of desperation.

Training

Training your team does not need to be complicated, but it should be a mandatory step in your staff onboarding. Aside from having your staff complete the necessary new hire paperwork, you should always dedicate sufficient time and budget to training.

For massage therapists and receptionist positions, two to three days is usually enough. Managers and leads may need more time to learn their job role. To many, this sounds extreme and expensive. However, this avoids the accusation of never being shown how to perform a task or that a staff member was not aware of what their responsibilities were.

Begin by organizing how your staff will be trained. This can be achieved by creating a 1-2 page bullet point of their responsibilities within your operating procedures starting before the beginning of the client journey.

Before the client arrives at your massage facility, certain tasks need to be done. The appointment should have been confirmed. The facility should be clean. New client paperwork should be ready. Past client history should be reviewed. If you offer any amenities for clients prior to their service, everything should be prepared ahead of time so nothing cuts into their time. The treatment room should be set up based on the service they will be receiving. These are just a few tasks that need to be done consistently before the client shows up and someone has to be responsible for them. The responsible parties must be trained.

I've found that it is much easier to train staff in the order in which they will be performing tasks. This helps reinforce the importance of routine and how you prefer their job to be done. When a job feels like a routine your staff is less likely to skip steps or perform them at their own discretion. It is also easier for you to identify where a breakdown occurs if and when a complaint occurs.

If you find that your business is receiving numerous complaints about a specific staff member, this may be a sign that they were improperly trained or that they are performing the task to their discretion. Investigate the situation to discover the problem.

When your staff has completed their training, it is best to have them sign or initial each training section to indicate that they have been properly trained and have not questions. Future questions will arise. They may forget how to perform the task when they are left to work independently. Be understanding that some employees require a bit more practice before a task becomes routine. Gradually ease them into independence instead of assuming they have mastered their job after only a few days of training. This should be reasonable considering most massage therapists who start their business take months and even years before they consistently perform a service or task. It may take your staff a bit longer to learn new tasks. Some may need to break old habits they've been conditioned to perform at a previous employer. Exercising patience and displaying empathy can go a long way in showing your staff that they are appreciated and a valuable addition to your team.

The final step is assigning the task of training to someone. If you, the owner, will not be training your new staff, make sure to train your designated trainer. A common complaint within many businesses is not being trained properly. When this complaint is brought to the trainer, their response is they were never shown how. Never assume that just because someone knows how to do their job, they also possess the skills to train someone else.

Ask yourself:
Has my staff been trained?

____

____

____

Were expectations clearly articulated?

____

____

____

How long ago was my staff trained?

____

____

____

Have there been any significant changes in my business's operating procedures since their training?

____

____

____

If so, how were those changes communicated?

____

____

____

Have I updated my existing training procedures to include those changes?

____

____

____

How will I confirm that my staff has been trained?

____

____

____

How long does training last for each position?

____

____

____

Have I budgeted enough resources towards training? (Time and money)

____

____

____

How will my trainees be evaluated?

____

____

____

Do I have a designated "Trainer"?

____

____

____

Have I trained my "Trainer"?

____

____

____

Retention

If you have ever recruited or hired a staff member before, you already know how expensive it is to recruit and train new staff. It is much more cost effective to train and retain an existing staff member than it is to hire a new one. If you have existing staff that is not working out, this may be the time to review your training procedures.

It is just as important to follow up and gain feedback from employees as it is your clients. Too many businesses assume that staff will openly discuss their concerns with management when that is far from the truth. You may think that a quiet employee is content, when in fact they are ready to quit the moment they find a new or better opportunity.

When an employee quits, it causes significant financial strain on a massage business. Clients grow attached to their therapists. And while the massage service is not the only reason a client chooses to remain loyal to a business, it does weigh heavily in their decision.

When a massage business loses an employee, they lose money in recruitment, training and revenue from the clients who refuse to schedule with anyone else. In addition, the business appears to be unstable from a client and employee perspective. This makes it more challenging to recruit good staff.

Good employees tend to recommend your business to their colleagues. They also advertise their place of employment to their existing client base. This helps the business save on advertising costs across the board.

So how do you as an owner retain these great employees? You get to know your team on a personal level. Spend some time learning what motivates them. Discover what they love about their current work environment. Allow them the freedom to openly discuss what they don't like without the threat of punishment or retaliation. Provide a safe and anonymous way for them to express concerns and offer feedback. Dedicate consistent one on one time with your staff to learn about their future goals and suggestions for how you could improve your business. Allow yourself to be transparent.

Many business owners avoid opening themselves or their business up to their employees. The reason most likely is due to lack of trust. If you are going to hire employees, there needs to be a certain level of trust in both directions. You need to trust that your employees will not steal or share your trade secrets and client information. Your employees need to trust that they will be paid on time and treated with respect. While these seem like reasonable and minimal expectations, the sad truth is many employers and employees find themselves in situations that fall short.

We have already discussed in a quite a bit of detail a few ways in which an employer can retain good staff. Providing great benefits, communicating responsibilities and expectations, training to standards and procedures, dedicating time to get to know your staff personally, and providing a frequent and safe space for feedback.

What other steps can you actively take to retain your staff? If you are having trouble with identifying steps you as the owner can take, review your own list of reasons you chose to start your business. There is a good chance one of the reasons had to do with your past or current employer.

If you currently have employees, this is a great time to ask for feedback and genuinely listen. You'll discover that salary will rarely come up in the conversation. This is because your staff is made aware of what their starting salary will be prior to accepting the job.

If they remain unhappy with their salary, you may need to consider offering a wage increase to those staff members who have been loyal and to those who have gone above and beyond what is expected of them.

Consider scheduling regular objective evaluations. Publicly acknowledge the employees who excel at their job. Recognition goes a long way in building loyalty and highlighting acceptable behavior you want your employees to emulate. Other employees should see that good behavior is appreciated and rewarded.

If you have never had employees, this is a great place to start. Use the space below to list the ways your previous employer could have kept you.

6 METRICS AND KPIS

Analyzing data can be a snooze. Especially when you don't know what to look for or what the data means in regards to your business. This section is important because you cannot improve your performance if it is not measured. If performance is going to be measured then it should be monitored and managed as well. In this section, we will identify relevant metrics, provide tips on how to set benchmarks and offer advice on what actions to take if your results begin to stray.

Every owner should analyze their business's performance frequently. Qualitative analysis is generally performed through client and employee feedback and reviews. It can also be obtained by hiring secret shoppers who evaluate your business objectively. Quantitative analysis is another form of insight that is often neglected, especially when your business is young.

Many new owners limit their quantitative analysis to

reviewing revenue, expenses and profit margins. However there are many other numbers that tell a much deeper story. I strongly believe it benefits every business owner to understand how to evaluate their business both qualitatively and quantitatively. Because quantitative analysis possesses a bit of subjectivity and varies depending on how an owner has chosen to operate their business, this book will not cover that method of evaluation. Quantitative analysis is objective and relies on real numbers. The results are not subjective.

Let's begin by stating the difference between metrics and key performance indicators (KPIs). Some analysts use the terms interchangeably, but they are not the same.

A KPI can be a metric, but a metric is not necessarily a KPI. Metrics are simple numbers, while KPIs are statistics that give insight into how your massage business is performing.

Here is an example to help clarify the difference between a metric and a KPI. You are exploring ways to increase monthly revenue in your massage business. You believe your business could make more money if you had more upsells to advanced treatments. However, you can't *improve* this area in your business if you have not measured it to begin with. First, you'll need to know your current upsell percentage. This number is obtained by dividing the total number of upgrades you have sold by the total number of treatments sold in a given period of time. The result of that calculation is your upsell percentage. The total number of upgrades is a metric. The total number of treatments sold is a metric. The upgrade percentage is a KPI that assesses how efficient your staff is at sales.

Now that you have a good idea of the difference

between metrics and KPIs, lets explore the necessary metrics and top 10 relevant KPIs in a massage business.

Necessary Metrics

Your metrics are not difficult to locate or calculate. They are used in conjunction with the KPIs in the next section. You may have more metrics that you choose to measure or focus on. Depending on your goals or the information you need, you may choose to track many different metrics for a given period of time.

For example, during the holiday season, you may want to sell more gift certificates than the previous year. Unless you know how many you sold last year, you will not be able to set a realistic goal for the upcoming year.

1. **Total Revenue**

    Your total revenue accounts for all your business income. This includes retail, memberships, gift certificates, etc.

2. **Total Massage Revenue**

    Your total treatment revenue is only for revenue generated from massage treatments. Do not include retail.

3. **Total Operating Expenses**

    Your total operating expenses include everything

related to your massage business's core operations. This includes things like payroll, commissions, transportation, rent, supplies, repairs, taxes, etc. It does not include depreciation, amortization, interest charges or other costs of borrowing.

4. Gross Operating Profit

Your gross operating profit is the amount that is left over after subtracting your total revenue from your total operating expenses.

5. Total Number Of Clients

The total number of clients that were treated in a given period.

6. Number Of New Clients

The number of new clients treated in a given period.

7. Number Of Re-Booked Clients

The number of clients who rescheduled immediately after their session.

8. Number Of Repeat Clients

The number of clients treated in a given period that are not new.

9. Total Available Operating Hours

The total available hours of operation.

10. Total Massage Hours Available

Total number of massage treatment hours available. This number is based on the number of tables in your practice.

11. Total Massage Room Hours Available

Total number of treatment room hours available. This number is based on the number of treatment rooms in your practice.

12. Total Massage Hours Sold

This is the total number of HOURS sold. This may or may not be equivalent to the total number of treatments sold.

13. Total Upgraded Sessions

The total number of upgraded or advanced services. Typically this would be services like aromatherapy, hot stones, deep tissue, etc. They are counted if your business charges more for the session. If whatever upgrade you offer is already included in the standard service, do not count it as an upgrade.

14. Total Massage Hours Staffed

This is the total number of hours your massage team was scheduled. This may or may not be equivalent to the total number of treatment hours sold.

Relevant KPIs

The following top 10 KPIs are what I consider the most relevant ones to track for your massage business. There may be some you believe are not relevant to your practice. In that case, you can choose to ignore them. But having a good understanding of these metrics will help you pinpoint what is happening in your business at a glance.

1. Average Client Spend

Total Revenue / Total Number of Clients

This KPI measures the average amount that clients spend per visit. The most important variable in this KPI is the price of your services. You can increase your average client spend by:

- Increasing your menu prices
- Upsell add ons, advanced sessions, packages or retail
- Remove low cost services from your menu
- Eliminate discounts or deals

2. Average Session Length

Total Session Hours Sold / Total Number of Sessions

This KPI indicates whether you are only selling general sessions basic services or packages and sessions at longer lengths. The most important variable in this KPI is the length of sessions you have on your menu. You can improve your average session length by:

- Adding longer sessions to your menu
- Removing shorter sessions from your menu
- Upselling longer sessions
- Sell packages

3. Re-booking Rate

Number of Clients Who Re-book / Total Number of Clients

This KPI tracks the percentage of clients who re-book immediately after their treatment. A high rebooking percentage is a great indicator that clients are satisfied with their service. For this KPI, ONLY count clients who re-book immediately after their session, not later in the future. That metric can be captured in a different KPI. You can improve your re-book rate by:

- Incentivizing re-booking for both clients and staff
- Create a script that your staff can follow to improve re-booking
- Improve your service standards and procedures
- Provide clients with written recommendations of when to return
- Offer a small complimentary gift following each appointment

4. Upsell Rate

Number of Session Upgrades / Total Number of Sessions Sold

This KPI measures how effectively you and your team can sell. Upgrades can be sold by anyone on the staff, not just the front desk. They can be sold before and even during the start of the session. Your upsell rate can be improved by:

- Training your staff so they are all comfortable selling upgrades
- Offering a script for upsells
- Incentivizing upsell performance
- Offering a small menu of upgrade options in the treatment room
- Requiring each staff member to make at least one upsell attempt

- Providing recognition to top sellers on your team

5. Repeat Client Percentage

Number of Repeat Clients / Total Clients

This KPI is another measurement of client satisfaction. This KPI is similar to the Re-book rate, but includes clients who do not re-book immediately after their session. The repeat client percentage can be improved by:

- Following up with past clients
- Incentivizing future bookings
- Sending a personalized "thank you" card in the mail
- Selling packages
- Notifying past clients of current and future open appointments
- Actively engaging with past clients on social media
- Specifically targeting former clients in a marketing campaign

6. Service Capacity

Total Session Hours Sold / Total Massage Hours Available

This KPI lets you know how closely you are operating at full capacity. It is important to note that your available massage hours is based on the number of available massage tables you have, not just the number of rooms. That means if one of your treatment rooms has two tables and can accommodate couples massages, it counts as two available massage hours. In addition, if you have tables that are in a public or open space where you still treat clients, be sure to count those tables towards your available hours as well. You can improve your rate of occupancy by:

- Hiring more staff
- Shortening or adjusting your hours of operation
- Scheduling more couples massages (if applicable)
- Encouraging group bookings
- Increase or improve your marketing efforts
- Follow up with past clients
- Notify clients of current and future openings

7. Treatment Room Occupancy

Total Session Hours Sold / Total Massage Room Hours Available

This KPI tells you how busy your rooms are, but not your capacity. This is because some massage businesses have treatment rooms that hold two tables to accommodate a couple's massage. Those rooms can also be used to serve a single client. While that room is occupied, it is not operating at full capacity. You can improve your treatment room occupancy by:

- Hiring more staff
- Encouraging group bookings
- Increase or improve your marketing efforts
- Follow up with past clients
- Notify clients of current and future openings
- Shorten or adjust your hours of operation

8. Staffing Efficiency (Massage Therapists)

Total Massage Treatment Hours Performed / Total Massage Hours Scheduled

This KPI measures the productivity of your massage therapists in regards to performing services. More than likely, they do not schedule themselves so it is imperative that you or the scheduling manager pay close attention to this metric. If this number is consistently low, you may be overstaffed. If your number is too high, you may need to consider hiring more staff. Other ways you can improve your staffing efficiency is by:

- Improving service standards and policies

- Take steps to improve your re-booking rate
- Improve or increase your marketing efforts
- Adjust your hours of operation
- Notify clients of current or future openings
- Provide clients with written recommendations of when to return
- Adjust the staff schedule to reflect the amount of services for the day
- Offer staff the ability to work "on-call"

9. Revenue Efficiency

Total Massage Revenue / Total Massage Hours Available

This KPI indicates how efficient your massage business is in terms of generating revenue. This KPI, like the service capacity, take all the treatment tables into consideration, not just the treatment rooms. You can improve your revenue efficiency by:

- Scheduling more couple's massage
- Encouraging group bookings
- Minimizing discounts and deals
- Increasing service upgrades
- Hire more staff

- Offer shorter or mini services that may not require a private room

10. Gross Operating Efficiency

Total Gross Operating Profit / Total Massage Hours Available

This final KPI measures how efficient your entire massage business is operating. It is a great indicator of how well you generate revenue, control expenses and your profitability. You can improve your gross operating efficiency by:

- Minimizing product waste
- Improving staffing efficiency
- Increasing your average client spend
- Minimizing discounts and deals
- Increasing upsells and upgrades
- Increasing re-book rate
- Improving your staffing efficiency
- Increase your prices
- Get rid of unnecessary expenses
- Reevaluate the wages you pay and adjust if you are overpaying

Understanding what these numbers are, how they affect your business and the steps to take to improve performance is critical. That point cannot be overstated.

A question that comes up frequently is when to begin collecting this data. The answer is now! It is never too late and there is never a wrong time. You don't need to wait to the beginning of the month or year to start gathering this data.

If you are using a scheduling or payment software for your business, you can pull past numbers quickly. This task doesn't need to be daunting. Much of this information can be collected in less than an hour. It is well worth the time investment if it can lead to improving your future revenue and profits in the long run.

Using the next few pages you can begin tracking your data. For free printable templates, head over to:

www.spa-analytics.com/Free-Templates

Metrics

Month: _______________ Year: _________

Total Revenue	
Total # Of Clients	
Total # Of Session Hours Sold	
Total # Of Sessions Sold	
# Of Re-Books	
# Of Upgrades	
Total Session Hours	
# Of Repeat Clients	
# Of Massage Hours Available	
Total Room Hours Available	
# of Hours Scheduled	
Total Service Revenue	
Total Gross Operating Profit	

KPIs

Month: _____________ Year: _______

Average Client Spend	
Average Session Length	
Re-Booking Rate	
Upsell Rate	
Repeat Client Percentage	
Service Capacity	
Treatment Room Occupancy	
Staffing Efficiency	
Revenue Efficiency	
Gross Operating Efficiency	

SETTING BENCHMARKS AND GOALS

Your benchmarks and goals will be unique to you and your business. As emphasized throughout this book, no two businesses are alike. Unless you have invested in a franchise or turnkey massage business, you will need to create all of your own benchmarks and goals.

The first step, which hopefully you have completed in the previous section, is gathering your past data. Ideally, you will want to track your data monthly. Gather as much information as far back as you can go. If your business is not new, hopefully you can gather data from at least the past 12 months. 24 months would be optimal.

After you've gathered the data, you will need to review it. Take note of any obvious trends. Because the massage industry has a tendency to experience seasonal highs and lows, you may notice inconsistencies in data during those times. If there are other time periods or certain months where your numbers seemed extraordinarily high or low, make a note of it. It could be that you changed locations, hired more staff, or invested in a new marketing effort. You want to be able to explain any anomalies in your data.

Using your past data, you can begin to see averages. That is why it is ideal to have data from at least 24 months before you begin to set goals. If you are new to business or simply do not have all the data, you can still just use the information you have. You just may risk setting goals and benchmarks that are too high or too low. You can always adjust them over time.

Based on your average numbers, you can set *reasonable* benchmarks for where your numbers *should* be. If over the past 6 month, you serve an average 10 new clients, that should be your benchmark for every month moving forward. If you experience more or less than that, you should be able to explain why. You may have seen less clients if you took a week vacation. You may have seen less clients if one of your massage therapists quit. Conversely, you may have seen more new clients if you hired a new staff member or extended your operating hours.

If the reason you experienced a difference above or below the benchmark is permanent, you want to adjust the benchmark to reflect that. If the reason for the difference is only temporary, simply make a note of why, and keep your benchmark the same.

How often you review your data is up to you. You may choose to only review your numbers quarterly or annually. There is no right or wrong way. The key is to be consistent in whatever method or approach you use. Reviewing your information too frequently can be just as damaging as not reviewing often enough. This is because some changes you apply need time to take affect.

If you don't have enough data because you haven't been in business long or you believe your numbers are still too low, you will not be able to set reasonable benchmarks. Instead, you will be setting goals based on what you *need* in order for your business to be sustainable.

To set these goals, begin by identifying all of your expenses. If your business is also meant to support your personal expenses, make sure you include all those expenses as well. Use that amount to create your revenue goals. From there, you can break down how you believe you can achieve that goal. You may choose to start with a set number of clients per month. After that, you may set upgrade goals to help increase your revenue. You may also focus increasing the number of gift card or package sales. As you get busier, you may hire a staff member to help you achieve those revenue goals.

If you are already in business and have stable benchmarks but are trying to improve or grow your business, you will need to set new goals as well. Let's assume you reviewed your data over the past 4 years and noticed that during the holiday season you sell an average of 400 gift certificates. Your goal this year may be to sell 500. If this is a goal you decide to set, you want to first acknowledge how you have been able to achieve the 400 in the first place. Decide what you can do differently to attract an extra 100 sales. This may be offering a gift card deal, beginning your holiday promotions sooner, or deploying a completely new marketing effort in addition to the ones you've done before. Maybe you want to offer a sales incentive to motivate your team.

When you set goals, create a plan for how you will achieve them. Make your entire staff aware of your business goals, their responsibilities as it pertains to achieving them and how they benefit from reaching or exceeding that goal. Give yourself and your business enough time to plan and execute. Waiting one week before the holidays to start planning will yield poor results and demoralize you and the team.

The sooner you can begin creating benchmarks, setting new goals, and planning your execution, the better chance your business has at development and growth. If you have found yourself falling into the trap of last minute planning and marketing efforts, try keeping a business calendar or journal. Begin planning at least a quarter (3 months) in advance. When it's time to execute you and your team are not overwhelmed with the process.

7 WHAT NOW?

I hope that once you've finished reading and working through this book that you are able to see your business as an entity that can function without you. It is unreasonable to suggest that you can go immediately from outlining your operations to flipping a switch and stepping out of your treatment room in a single day. The point is to show you it is possible and you too can create a business that is a well oiled wheel if you are clear on what and how you do things. You are aware that focusing on intangible details that are just as important as the things you can hold in your hand or see in front of you.

To recap, we've discussed how to effectively communicate with your ideal client. You have identified a real problem your ideal client is facing. You understand how your services solve that problem. And you have created an amazing offer to attract those clients to your business.

You have expressed the reasons you chose to go into business for yourself and how those reasons are at the forefront of how you treat your clients and staff. Those priorities were then used as guidelines to create your service standards and policies to support them.

We then took a quick tour of the client's journey and identified some of the critical touch points. From there you were able to begin outlining your operations from the time your client arrives to the time they leave. You should have been able specify how certain tasks would be performed, who is responsible and what policies you will create to ensure your operating standards are met. By breaking the client journey into manageable pieces, you felt less overwhelmed and could easily see how to develop and build your operating procedures.

Later we discussed the importance of recruiting, training and retaining your ideal staff. Combining your reasons for starting your own business, your standards and operating procedures, you were able to identify who you need on staff, what you would like to pay, and the qualifications you are seeking in an ideal candidate.

After identifying your necessary staff, you outlined how you would train them, how you would establish accountability, measure performance and some things you could do to retain them for the long run. Arguably, you have no control over whether a staff member chooses to stay or go. But as owner, you need to be aware of your company culture and keep the lines of communication open with everyone involved in your business.

Finally, we covered one of the most daunting parts of your massage business. You were able to define, track and measure metrics and key performance indicators that are relevant to the massage industry. You received tips on how to manage each of those numbers and what to do if you fall below. You also were able to create benchmarks and goals based on your past performance or future predictions.

You are aware there is much more to running a business than what I have covered in this book. No single book can replace the knowledge you will gain through trial and error. Please take what you have learned and worked on throughout this book and apply it. There is no value if information is only consumed and never put to use.

Good luck with building your massage business! For more business tips and resources, head over to www.spa-analytics.com.

ABOUT THE AUTHOR

Kamillya Hunter is a former massage therapist and self-diagnosed spa junkie. She is the owner of Spa Analytics, a consulting firm that focuses on strengthening independently owned spa and massage businesses. She is also the national best selling author of Success Of A Failed Therapist and Touched: True Stories From Inside The Massage Room. For more resources, check out www.spa-analytics.com

Other books by Kamillya Hunter:

Success Of A Failed Therapist

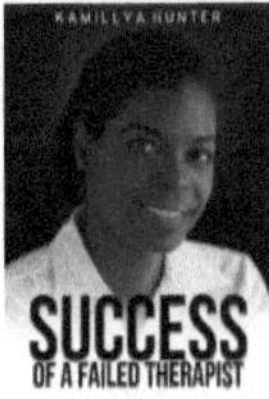

Touched: True Stories From Inside The Massage Room

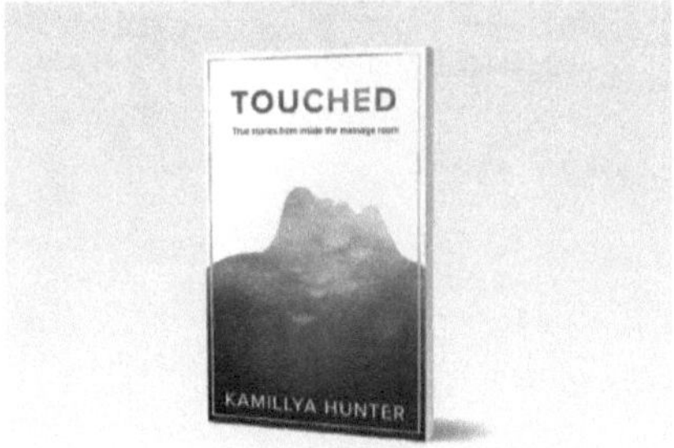